GALLBLADDER PAIN

GREAT REMEDIES FOR GALLBLADDER PAIN

DR. J. WALLER

Contents

Introduction

Generally speaking, gallbladder pain refers to discomfort or pain brought on by problems with the gallbladder, a little organ situated under the liver. Because it stores and secretes bile, a fluid that facilitates the breakdown of fats, the gallbladder is an essential component of the digestive system. This is a quick overview of gallbladder pain:

Where the Gallbladder Is:

On the right side of the belly, below the liver, is where the gallbladder is located. It is connected to the small intestine and liver via a network of ducts.

Storage and Release of Bile:

Bile produced by the liver is stored in the gallbladder. The gallbladder contracts during digestion, particularly after eating fatty foods, and discharges bile into the small intestine to help break down fats.

Gallbladder Pain Causes:

A number of conditions, such as gallstones, inflammation (cholecystitis), infections, or other problems impairing the gallbladder's regular operation, can cause gallbladder pain.

Gallstones:

Solid particles called gallstones develop in the gallbladder. They may cause pain, particularly when the gallbladder contracts, and obstruct the regular flow of bile.

Cholecystitis:

Cholecystitis, or gallbladder inflammation, can be painful and uncomfortable. This inflammation could be long-term or short-term.

Gallbladder Pain Symptoms:

Upper right abdominal discomfort that feels acute or crampy is a common symptom of gallbladder pain. The right shoulder or back may also feel the ache. Bloating in the abdomen, nausea, and vomiting are possible additional symptoms.

Factors that aggravating and triggering:

Eating fatty or oily foods might cause or worsen gallbladder pain. Consuming these meals can cause the gallbladder to contract, which, if there are underlying problems, can cause pain.

Diagnostic Examinations:

Medical practitioners can determine the origin of gallbladder pain by a variety of diagnostic procedures, including blood tests, CT scans, and ultrasounds.

Options for Treatment:

The fundamental reason determines the treatment strategy. Certain situations may call for the recommendation of drugs, dietary adjustments, or lifestyle changes. A cholecystectomy, or surgical removal of the gallbladder, is a popular treatment for serious or persistent conditions.

People who have severe or chronic stomach discomfort, particularly on the right side, should consult a doctor so they may get a proper diagnosis and evaluation. The severity of gallbladder discomfort can vary, and it may be a sign of underlying problems that need to be treated by a doctor.

CHAPTER ONE

Structure and Purpose of the Gallbladder

The gallbladder is a little, pear-shaped organ that is situated in the upper abdomen of the right side, beneath the liver. By collecting and releasing bile, a digestive fluid the liver produces, it plays a critical function in digestion. Let's examine the gallbladder's structure and operation:

The gallbladder's anatomy:

Where:

On the right side of the belly, below the liver, is where the gallbladder is located.

Dimensions and Form:

Its form is pear-shaped, and its length ranges from 3 to 4 inches.

Links:

The hepatic duct connects the gallbladder to the liver, and the common bile duct connects it to the small intestine, more especially the duodenum.

Organization:

The fundus (base), body, and neck make up the gallbladder. It contains a muscular wall that enables it to contract and release bile, and it is lined with a mucous membrane.

What the Gallbladder Does

The main job of the gallbladder is to hold and expel bile, a digestive juice that facilitates fat absorption and digestion. There are multiple steps in the process:

Production of Bile:

Bile is continuously produced by the liver. Water, bile salts, cholesterol, bilirubin, and other chemicals make up bile.

Bile Reserve:

The gallbladder holds on to bile after it leaves the liver through the hepatic ducts and is used for storage during meals. Bile is concentrated and stored in the gallbladder until it is required for digestion, serving as a reservoir.

Bile Expulsion:

The gallbladder contracts and releases bile into the small intestine through the common bile duct when a person eats, particularly if the meal contains lipids.

Facilitating Digestion:

Fats get emulsified by bile and are broken down into tiny droplets. This procedure helps the small intestine's enzymes break down lipids more thoroughly.

Absorption of Nutrients:

The process by which fatty acids and fat-soluble vitamins (A, D, E, and K) are absorbed from the digestive system into the bloodstream depends heavily on bile.

Hormonal signals, including cholecystokinin (CCK), are responsible for the gallbladder's contraction. CCK is released when fats are present in the small intestine.

The gallbladder aids in digesting, however it is not necessary for life. A cholecystectomy, or surgical removal of the gallbladder, can be done if necessary without having a major effect on digestion, but dietary changes could be advised.

Gallbladder Pain Factors

There are several reasons for gallbladder discomfort, most of which have to do with problems that interfere with the gallbladder's regular operation. The following are typical reasons for gallbladder pain:

Cholelithiasis, or gallstones:

Solid particles called gallstones develop in the gallbladder. They may obstruct the bile's regular flow, causing pain and suffering. When the gallbladder contracts in an effort to discharge bile, discomfort may be experienced.

Cholecystitis:

Cholecystitis, or gallbladder inflammation, is a condition that can hurt. Infections or gallstones obstructing the bile ducts may be the cause of this inflammation.

Biliary Colic:

Gallstones that temporarily clog the cystic duct are the source of sporadic and recurrent episodes of discomfort associated with biliary colic.

Gallbladder dysfunction (Biliary dyskinesia):

An inability of the gallbladder to contract and release bile in a normal manner can result in pain and discomfort.

Choledocholithiasis:

Gallstones have the potential to go into the common bile duct, obstructing it and producing discomfort. Choledocholithiasis is the name given to this illness.

Gallbladder Polyps:

Small growths called polyps on the gallbladder wall can hurt, particularly if they obstruct bile flow or become inflammatory.

Gallbladder Mucus:

A thicker mixture of bile constituents that can build up in the gallbladder is referred to as sludge. It could result in pain and suffering akin to that brought on by gallstones.

Disorder of the Functional Gallbladder:

Gallstones or inflammation may not be present in the gallbladder pain experienced by some people. We refer to this ailment as functional gallbladder disorder.

Injury or Trauma:

Gallbladder discomfort can be brought on by abdominal trauma, such as an injury or surgical procedure.

Growths:

Pain may result from tumors in the gallbladder or surrounding tissues, particularly if they block the bile flow.

Infections

Gallbladder infections are uncommon, although they can cause pain. Infection might happen as a result of systemic illnesses or gallstones.

Cast Iron Gallbladder:

Pain may occasionally result from the gallbladder wall being hardened, a condition known as porcelain gallbladder.

It's crucial to remember that gallbladder discomfort can range in severity and that certain foods, particularly fatty or greasy ones, might cause or worsen it. People who have severe or chronic stomach discomfort, especially on the right side, should consult a doctor so they can be properly evaluated and diagnosed.

Symptoms and Indications

There are many different indications and symptoms that can accompany gallbladder pain, and the severity of these symptoms can also vary. The following are typical indications and manifestations of gallbladder pain:

Pain in upper right abdomen:

Usually, the upper right quadrant of the abdomen, just behind the ribs, is where pain or discomfort is felt. Moreover, it could spread to the right shoulder blade or the back.

Sharp or Strangling Aches:

Many people describe the discomfort as agonizing, cramping, or acute. It could come and go, particularly after eating.

Pain Caused by Consuming Food:

Eating fatty or oily foods can frequently cause gallbladder pain. During digestion, the gallbladder contracts to release bile, and if there are underlying problems, this process may cause pain.

vomiting and nauseous:

Some people may feel sick to their stomachs and throw up, especially if the pain is really bad.

CHAPTER TWO

Achy in the abdomen:

Touching the area above the gallbladder may cause it to become painful, and applying pressure there may make the pain worse.

Bloating and Indigestion:

After eating, bloating, and a full feeling may be connected to symptoms of gallbladder pain.

Belching and Gas:

Gallbladder pain may also be accompanied by increased gas and burp.

Colds and fever:

When gallbladder inflammation (cholecystitis) is present, people may get chills and a temperature.

Greenish-white color:

Rarely, jaundice a yellowing of the skin and eyes may result from a gallstone obstructing the common bile duct.

Color Shifts in the Stool:

Pale or light-colored feces might occasionally be the result of gallbladder problems.

It's crucial to remember that although gallbladder discomfort is frequently brought on by particular triggers, such as meals, the symptoms can sometimes be vague and mimic those of other gastrointestinal disorders. Seeking early medical assistance is essential for a good evaluation and diagnosis if someone has severe or chronic stomach discomfort, especially on the right side. Imaging investigations or ultrasonography are examples of diagnostic tests that can be performed to find the underlying cause of the symptoms.

In order to determine the underlying cause of gallbladder discomfort, a combination of physical examination, medical history assessment, and diagnostic tests is usually used in the diagnosis and evaluation process. An outline of the procedure for diagnosing gallbladder pain is provided below:

Health Background:

The patient's medical history will be questioned by the healthcare professional, who will also want to know about the type and length of the pain, any related symptoms like nausea or vomiting, and triggers or aggravating foods.

Physical Assessment:

It is possible to perform a physical examination to check for any signs of discomfort, such as tenderness or swelling, in the abdomen. In addition, the medical professional might look for additional symptoms including jaundice.

Blood Examinations:

To evaluate liver function and look for indications of infection or inflammation, blood tests may be carried out. Increased bilirubin or liver enzyme levels could be a sign of gallbladder problems.

Imaging Research:

The gallbladder and associated components can be seen using a variety of imaging studies:

Ultrasound: This non-invasive imaging procedure creates images of the gallbladder by using sound waves. It may indicate the existence of inflammation, gallstones, or other anomalies.

CT Scan: To acquire precise cross-sectional images of the abdomen and aid in the diagnosis of gallbladder problems, a computed tomography (CT) scan may be carried out.

Hepatobiliary iminodiacetic acid (HIDA) scan: This nuclear medicine test assesses the gallbladder's health and can identify problems like blockage.

Endoscopic Examinations:

Endoscopic tests might be advised in certain circumstances:

Endoscopic Ultrasound (EUS): This method creates finely detailed pictures of the gallbladder and surrounding structures by combining endoscopy and ultrasound.

Endoscopic Retrograde Cholangiopancreatography (ERCP): This technique can be used to treat gallstones or other problems by seeing the bile ducts.

Cholecystogram:

During X-ray imaging, a cholecystogram uses contrast material to highlight the gallbladder.

Clinical Assessment:

When diagnosing a patient, the medical professional will take into account the patient's medical history, the severity of the symptoms, and the overall clinical presentation.

Appropriate treatment options can be considered after the underlying cause of gallbladder pain has been determined. This could involve dietary adjustments, pharmaceutical changes, lifestyle adjustments, or, in certain situations, surgery such a cholecystectomy to remove the gallbladder. For gallbladder-related problems to be effectively managed, an early and precise diagnosis is necessary.

Methods of Therapy

The underlying cause of gallbladder pain determines how best to treat it. The following are typical methods for treating gallbladder pain:

Modifications to Diet and Lifestyle:

It could be suggested to alter one's diet to treat gallbladder discomfort. This sometimes entails avoiding or consuming less fatty or oily meals, as these can aggravate symptoms and cause gallbladder contractions. It might also be advantageous to eat smaller, more frequent meals.

Drugs:

Nonsteroidal anti-inflammatory medicines (NSAIDs), like ibuprofen, are examples of pain management medications that may be prescribed to treat pain and reduce inflammation. Medication that dissolves gallstones may be taken into consideration in certain situations.

Handling of Supporting Conditions:

It is important to treat any underlying disorders that may be the source of gallbladder pain, such as gallstones or cholecystitis. For instance, if gallstones are present, treatment options can include the surgical removal of the gallbladder (cholecystectomy) or the use of drugs to dissolve the stones.

Antibiotics:

Antibiotics may be used to treat cholecystitis, if gallbladder inflammation is the result of an infection.

Pain Control:

Apart from non-steroidal anti-inflammatory drugs (NSAIDs), other pain management tactics could involve employing analgesics or muscle relaxants to alleviate discomfort.

Treatment for Gallstone Dissolution:

Certain gallstones, especially cholesterol stones, can be dissolved with medications such as ursodeoxycholic acid (ursodiol). This method works better with smaller stones, but it's not for everyone.

Endoscopic Techniques:

Endoscopic techniques such as endoscopic retrograde cholangiopancreatography (ERCP) may be used to remove or dissolve gallstones when they are the cause of obstruction.

Cholecystectomy surgery:

A typical treatment for gallbladder pain is surgical removal of the gallbladder (cholecystectomy), particularly if the discomfort is severe, recurrent, or linked to gallstones or inflammation. Traditional open surgery or less invasive laparoscopic surgery can be used to accomplish this.

Alternative Medical Interventions:

Some people might look into complementary therapies like acupuncture, herbal remedies, or dietary supplements. Nonetheless, prior to attempting any alternative remedies, medical advice must be sought.

The underlying reason of gallbladder discomfort, the intensity of symptoms, and the patient's general health all play a role in the treatment decision. It's critical that people with severe or chronic gallbladder discomfort consult a doctor in order to receive an accurate diagnosis and customized therapy.

Nutritional Aspects

When it comes to treating gallbladder pain, diet is very important, particularly if gallstones or inflammation (cholecystitis) are the cause of the discomfort. The following food suggestions can help reduce gallbladder pain:

Diet Low in Fat:

Limit your intake of fat in your diet, especially saturated and trans fats. Meals high in fat might exacerbate symptoms and cause contractions of the gallbladder. Choose lean protein sources including fish, lentils, and skinless chicken.

Don't Eat Fried or Greasy Foods:

Eat less fried and oily meals because these can aggravate gallbladder pain. Alternatively, opt for culinary techniques like steaming, grilling, or baking.

Restrict dairy products:

Cutting back on high-fat dairy products may provide relief for some people. Select dairy products that are fat-free or low-fat.

Select Whole Grains:

Consume whole grains like oats, brown rice, and whole wheat bread in your diet. These offer minerals and fiber without adding too much fat.

Boost Your Fiber Consumption:

Aim for a diet high in fruits, vegetables, whole grains, and other sources of fiber. In addition to regulating digestion, fiber may help avoid constipation.

Drinking plenty of water

Drink lots of water to be well hydrated. Drinking enough water promotes digestive health in general and inhibits the production of concentrated bile.

Little, Regular Meals:

Consider eating smaller, more frequent meals throughout the day as an alternative to large ones. This strategy might lessen the gallbladder's burden.

Steer clear of rapid weight loss:

Fast weight reduction can raise the risk of gallstone formation, particularly when done through crash diets. If necessary, strive for lasting weight loss that is gradual.

Limit alcohol and caffeine:

For certain people, alcohol and caffeine might exacerbate gallbladder symptoms. Think about reducing or limiting your intake of alcoholic and caffeinated beverages.

Add Lean Proteins:

Pick lean protein sources like fish, tofu, skinless chicken, and legumes. Avoid high-fat cuts of meat and processed meats.

Be Mindful of Trigger Foods:

Pay attention to specific foods that trigger or worsen gallbladder pain in your case. This may vary among individuals, so it's essential to identify personal triggers.

It's crucial to note that dietary recommendations may vary based on individual circumstances and the underlying cause of gallbladder pain. It's advisable to consult with a healthcare professional or a registered dietitian for personalized dietary guidance tailored to your specific situation. In some cases, surgical removal of the gallbladder (cholecystectomy) may be recommended, and dietary adjustments may be necessary post-surgery.

Coping Strategies and Lifestyle Modifications

Coping with gallbladder pain involves adopting lifestyle modifications and strategies to manage symptoms and improve overall well-being. Here are coping strategies for individuals experiencing gallbladder pain:

Dietary Modifications:

Follow a low-fat diet to minimize gallbladder contractions. Focus on lean proteins, whole grains, fruits, and vegetables. Avoid trigger foods that worsen symptoms.

Drink lots of water to be well hydrated. Proper hydration supports digestion and helps prevent the formation of concentrated bile.

Little, Regular Meals:

Instead of large meals, opt for smaller, more frequent meals throughout the day. This can reduce the workload on the gallbladder.

Steer clear of rapid weight loss:

If weight loss is a goal, aim for gradual and sustainable methods. Rapid weight loss can increase the risk of gallstone formation.

Regular Physical Activity:

Engage in regular physical activity, such as walking, swimming, or low-impact exercises. Physical activity can aid digestion and contribute to overall health.

Handling Stress:

Practice stress-reducing techniques such as deep breathing, meditation, or yoga. Stress can exacerbate digestive symptoms, including gallbladder pain.

Pain Control:

Use over-the-counter pain relievers, as recommended by a healthcare professional, to manage pain during episodes. Follow proper dosing instructions.

Hot Compress or Heating Pad:

Applying a hot compress or heating pad to the abdominal area may provide relief from muscle tension and discomfort.

Maintain a Food Journal:

Keep a food journal to track your diet and symptoms. This can help identify specific trigger foods that contribute to gallbladder pain.

Sleep Hygiene:

Prioritize good sleep hygiene by establishing a regular sleep routine. A well-rested body is better equipped to cope with pain and stress.

Educate Yourself:

Learn more about your condition and the factors that contribute to gallbladder pain.

Understanding your situation can empower you to make informed decisions about lifestyle changes.

Assist Mechanism:

Seek support from friends, family, or support groups. Sharing your experiences and feelings with others who understand can provide emotional support.

Consult with Healthcare Professionals:

Keep regular appointments with healthcare professionals to monitor your condition and discuss any changes in symptoms. Open communication is crucial for effective management.

It's important to note that coping strategies may vary among individuals, and what works for one person may not work for another. Consult with healthcare professionals, including a gastroenterologist and dietitian, to create a personalized plan tailored to your specific needs and circumstances. In some cases, surgical intervention, such as gallbladder removal (cholecystectomy), may be recommended for long-term relief.

CHAPTER THREE

Complications and Long-Term Effects

Gallbladder pain, if left untreated or associated with specific conditions, can lead to complications and potential long-term effects. Here are some complications and consequences of untreated or severe gallbladder pain:

Gallstones:

Untreated gallbladder pain, especially if caused by gallstones, can lead to complications such as cholecystitis (inflammation of the gallbladder), choledocholithiasis (obstruction of the common bile duct), and pancreatitis.

Cholecystitis:

Persistent gallbladder pain may result in recurrent or chronic inflammation of the gallbladder (cholecystitis), which can lead to complications like infection, abscess formation, or a perforated gallbladder.

Biliary Colic:

Recurrent episodes of biliary colic, characterized by severe pain due to gallstone obstruction, can impact the quality of life and lead to frequent discomfort.

Complications in Pregnancy:

Gallbladder issues during pregnancy, if left untreated, can pose risks to both the mother and the fetus. It may lead to complications such as cholecystitis or gallstone pancreatitis.

Long-Term Effects of Gallbladder Pain:

Postcholecystectomy Syndrome:

After gallbladder removal (cholecystectomy), some individuals may experience persistent symptoms, known as postcholecystectomy syndrome. This can include abdominal pain, bloating, and changes in bowel habits.

Digestive Changes:

Gallbladder removal can affect the digestion of fats. Some individuals may experience difficulty digesting fatty foods, leading to diarrhea or loose stools.

Bile Duct Issues:

Gallbladder pain, if associated with bile duct obstruction or inflammation, can lead to long-term issues with the bile ducts. This may include the formation of bile duct stones or strictures.

Sphincter of Oddi Dysfunction:

Dysfunction of the sphincter of Oddi, the muscular valve that controls the flow of bile and pancreatic juices, may persist after gallbladder removal, leading to pain and digestive issues.

Digestive Disorders:

Chronic gallbladder pain or complications may contribute to the development of digestive disorders, such as irritable bowel syndrome (IBS) or functional dyspepsia.

Gallbladder Cancer:

In rare cases, long-standing gallbladder issues, particularly if associated with chronic inflammation, may increase the risk of developing gallbladder cancer.

It's important to note that the severity of complications and long-term effects can vary among individuals. Timely medical intervention and appropriate treatment, including surgical removal of the gallbladder when necessary, are crucial for preventing or minimizing these complications. If you experience persistent or severe gallbladder pain, it's essential to seek medical attention for a thorough evaluation and appropriate management. Regular follow-up with healthcare professionals is recommended to monitor post-treatment recovery and address any concerns.

Postoperative Care and Recovery

Postoperative care and recovery after gallbladder removal (cholecystectomy) are essential for a smooth healing process and the prevention of complications. Here are key aspects of postoperative care and recovery:

1. Hospital Stay:

Cholecystectomy is commonly performed as a minimally invasive laparoscopic procedure, allowing for a shorter hospital stay compared to open surgery. Most patients can expect to go home on the same day or the day after surgery.

2. Pain Control:

Pain at the incision sites is common after surgery. Pain medications prescribed by the healthcare provider should be taken as directed to manage discomfort. Over-the-counter pain relievers may also be recommended.

3. Incision Care:

Follow proper incision care instructions provided by the healthcare team. Keep the incision sites clean and dry, and avoid exposing them to excessive moisture.

4. Activity and Rest:

While it's essential to avoid strenuous activities initially, gentle movements and walking can promote circulation and aid in recovery. Gradually increase activity levels as advised by the healthcare provider. Adequate rest is crucial for healing.

5. Modifications to Diet:

In the initial days after surgery, a temporary adjustment to a low-fat diet may be recommended to ease digestion. Slowly reintroduce regular foods as tolerated. Stay well-hydrated to prevent constipation.

6. Follow-Up Appointments:

Attend all scheduled follow-up appointments with the surgeon. These appointments allow for the monitoring of recovery progress, assessment of incisions, and addressing any concerns or questions.

7. Gradual Return to Normal Activities:

Return to normal activities, including work and daily routines, should be gradual. The timeline for resuming specific activities will depend on the individual's recovery and the type of surgery performed.

8. Signs of Complications:

Be vigilant for signs of complications, such as infection (redness, swelling, or discharge at incision sites), persistent pain, fever, or unusual symptoms. Report any concerns promptly to the healthcare provider.

9. Resuming Physical Activity:

Once cleared by the healthcare provider, gradually resume regular physical activity and exercise. Avoid heavy lifting or strenuous activities initially.

10. Dietary Considerations:

Resume a normal, balanced diet as tolerated. Most individuals do not require significant dietary restrictions after gallbladder removal.

11. Emotional Well-Being:

Surgery and recovery can be emotionally challenging. Seek support from friends, family, or a healthcare professional if needed. Be patient with the recovery process.

12. Driving Restrictions:

Follow any recommendations regarding driving restrictions postoperatively. It's typically advised to avoid driving until pain and discomfort are manageable, and you can perform emergency maneuvers comfortably.

13. Medication Management:

Take prescribed medications as directed, including any antibiotics or pain relievers. Inform the healthcare provider of any allergies or adverse reactions to medications.

Always follow the specific postoperative care instructions provided by the healthcare team. Individual recovery experiences may vary, and the healthcare provider will tailor recommendations based on the patient's unique circumstances. If any concerns or complications arise during the recovery period, promptly contact the healthcare provider for guidance.

CONCLUSION

In conclusion, gallbladder pain is often associated with conditions such as gallstones, inflammation (cholecystitis), or other issues affecting the gallbladder. The severity and frequency of pain can vary, and it's crucial to seek medical attention for a proper diagnosis and tailored treatment plan.

For those with gallbladder pain, lifestyle modifications, dietary changes, and, in some cases, surgical intervention may be recommended to manage symptoms effectively. Timely medical intervention is essential to address underlying causes, prevent complications, and improve overall well-being.

Postoperative care and recovery following gallbladder removal (cholecystectomy) play a vital role in ensuring a smooth healing process. Adhering to healthcare provider recommendations, managing pain appropriately, and gradually resuming normal activities contribute to a successful recovery.

It's important for individuals experiencing gallbladder pain to actively participate in their healthcare journey, communicate openly with healthcare professionals, and seek support from friends and family. Regular follow-up appointments and a proactive approach to health can contribute to a positive outcome.

As with any medical condition, individual experiences may vary, and personalized care is key. If you have concerns about gallbladder pain or are undergoing treatment, consult with your healthcare provider for guidance tailored to your specific needs. Overall, a proactive and informed approach to gallbladder health can lead to improved quality of life and well-being.

THE END

www.ingramcontent.com/pod-product-compliance
Lightning Source LLC
Chambersburg PA
CBHW060811260726

48660CB00002B/880